How to Use This Book

Once upon a Medical/Surgical ward in a hospital near you, a Registered Nurse precepted countless nursing students and noticed a common problem throughout entire cohorts of nearby programs.

Intelligent, book-smart students seemed to lack an understanding of how all of the concepts they had learned fit together. Each piece of information taught in nursing school is an important piece of a puzzle.

Concept maps are one of the best ways to study how information fits together. But concept maps are time-consuming to create and fill with information... right?

Introducing **The Med/Surg Mapper Workbook,** a color-coordinated workbook of concept map templates to assist in studying large amounts of information and memorizing the most pertinent facts and figures.

Ideally, use this workbook either before or after class to fill out information in every box. Not all diseases and conditions have a surgical intervention, so it's okay to specify "N/A" when this is true.

Filling out concept maps for the disease processes being covered in lecture *before* you attend class allows you to highlight the information that your professors emphasize during class, which could help you during your next exam.

Alternatively, filling out the concept maps *after* class facilitates a thorough review of each disease process before the exam, which can be equally beneficial in terms of memorizing information.

Because each type of information (i.e., etiology, symptoms, labs...) is present in the same place on each page, this workbook streamlines the process of flipping through pages of information before an exam to easily pick out the *unique* data specific to a certain disease.

To expand on that concept, there are many diseases characterized by fatigue and resulting in an elevated white blood cell count. But which diseases cause the patient to experience hyperactivity? What about hypocalcemia? How many diseases cause bradycardia *vs.* tachycardia?

Fill out the table of contents on Page 3 as you go for ease of looking up the maps you worked so hard to create. Utilize the blank pages in the back of the book for drawing your own, or capturing concepts that don't easily fit into the colored templates.

Pro tip, from someone who's been through it: invest in multi-colored pens and highlighters. Use one color for notes taken during independent study and another color of ink for information presented in class. Then have a highlighter to mark the content that was emphasized in class so you know where to focus for the exam.

Med/surg classes are no easy feat. Then again, you are not just an average nursing student. You have the passion, intelligence, and commitment to conquer nursing school. Let **The Med/Surg Master Mapper Workbook** help you in your journey.

~Lena Empyema

ASSESSMENT

Observable Signs:

* Jaundice
* Peri-umbilical gray/blue discoloration (Cullen's sign)
* If bleeding present:
  o Hypotension
  o Tachycardia
* Fever
* Decreased bowel sounds
* Weight loss

Subjective Symptoms.

* LUQ pain!! (most common)
  o Tender to palpation
* Nausea/vomiting
* Anorexia
* Diahrrea
* Malaise

HISTORY

Etiology:

Unknown in 20% of cases

Up to 90% of cases have gallstones blocking pancreatic ducts

Risk Factors:

Alcoholism

Some medications

Post-op Care:

* Standard care of incisions
* Pain mgmt

DIAGNOSTICS

Imaging:

* CT with contrast to diagnose
* Ultrasound to determine cause
* ERCP to visualize ducts

Labs:

* Increased amylase and lipase
* Increased WBC
* Decreased serum Ca & Mag

Disease/Condition:

Acute Pancreatitis

One-sentence description in my own words: "Potentially <u>life-threatening</u> inflammation of the pancreas involving premature activation of digestive enzymes"

TAKE ACTION

Non-surgical Interventions:

* NPO in early stages
* Then, low fat, high carb meals
  o Avoid spices, alcohol, and caffeine

EMERGENCY INTERVENTIONS:

! Pancreatic hemorrhage, watch VS, notify HCP!!

! Paralytic ileus, requiring NG insertion!!

!

Pharmaceutical Treatments:

* Opioids for pain mgmt. & to decrease secretion of digestive enzymes by liver
* Antibiotics for necrotizing pancreatitis

Pre-op Care:

* NPO

Surgical Interventions:

* Usually not needed, unless a lap chole is necessary (if gallstones are cause)
* Possible removal of pseudocyst

TABLE OF CONTENTS

Study. Dominate. Repeat.

ASSESSMENT

Observable Signs:

Subjective Symptoms:

HISTORY

Etiology:

Risk Factors:

DIAGNOSTICS

Imaging:

Labs:

Disease/Condition:

One-sentence description in my own words:

TAKE ACTION

Non-surgical
Interventions:

EMERGENCY
INTERVENTIONS:

!

!

!

!

Pharmaceutical Treatments:

Pre-op Care:

Surgical Interventions:

Post-op Care:

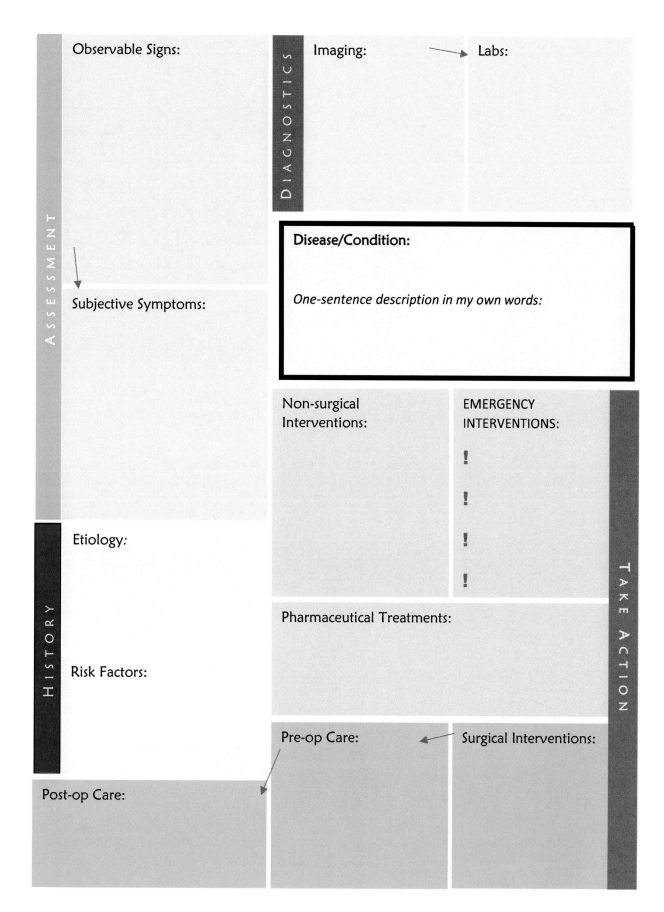

ASSESSMENT

Observable Signs:

Subjective Symptoms:

HISTORY

Etiology:

Risk Factors:

Post-op Care:

DIAGNOSTICS

Imaging:

Labs:

Disease/Condition:

One-sentence description in my own words:

Non-surgical
Interventions:

EMERGENCY
INTERVENTIONS:

!

!

!

!

Pharmaceutical Treatments:

Pre-op Care:

Surgical Interventions:

TAKE ACTION

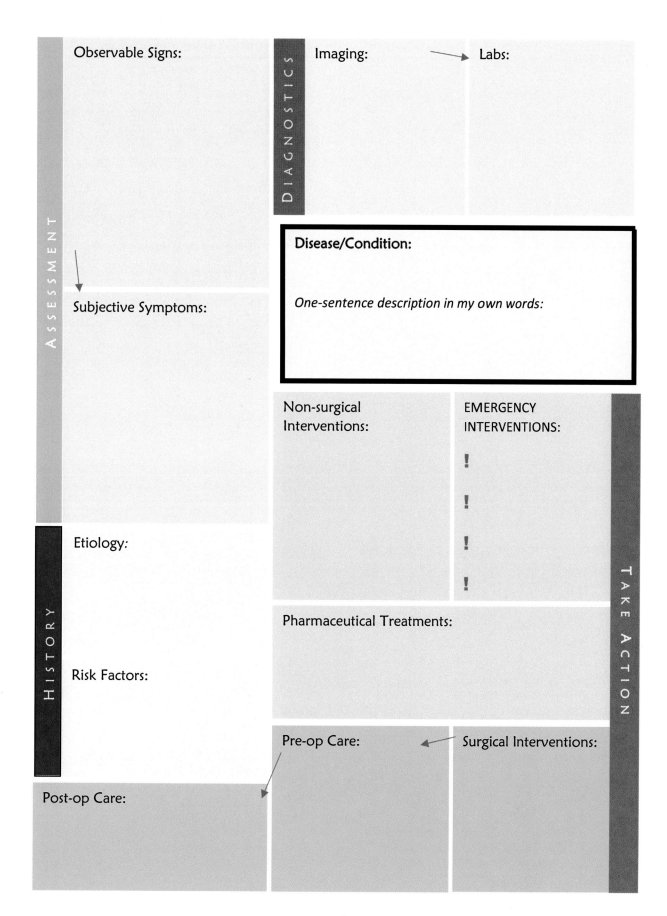

ASSESSMENT

Observable Signs:

Subjective Symptoms:

HISTORY

Etiology:

Risk Factors:

Post-op Care:

DIAGNOSTICS

Imaging:

Labs:

Disease/Condition:

One-sentence description in my own words:

Non-surgical Interventions:

EMERGENCY INTERVENTIONS:

!

!

!

!

Pharmaceutical Treatments:

Pre-op Care:

Surgical Interventions:

TAKE ACTION

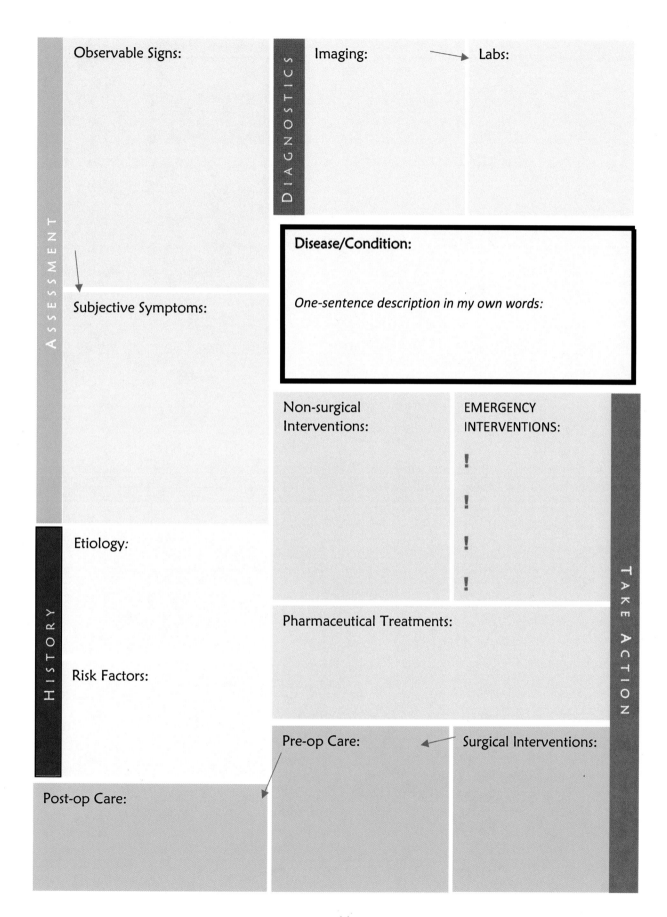

ASSESSMENT

Observable Signs:

Subjective Symptoms:

HISTORY

Etiology:

Risk Factors:

DIAGNOSTICS

Imaging:

Labs:

Disease/Condition:

One-sentence description in my own words:

Non-surgical Interventions:

EMERGENCY INTERVENTIONS:

!

!

!

!

Pharmaceutical Treatments:

Pre-op Care:

Surgical Interventions:

Post-op Care:

TAKE ACTION

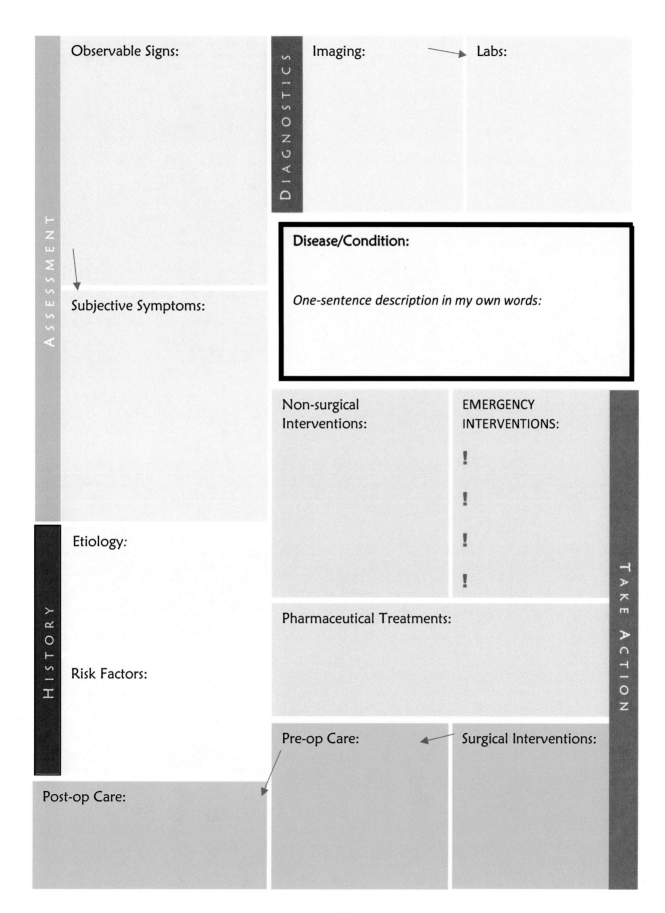

ASSESSMENT

Observable Signs:

Subjective Symptoms:

DIAGNOSTICS

Imaging:

Labs:

Disease/Condition:

One-sentence description in my own words:

HISTORY

Etiology:

Risk Factors:

Post-op Care:

Non-surgical Interventions:

EMERGENCY INTERVENTIONS:

!

!

!

!

Pharmaceutical Treatments:

Pre-op Care:

Surgical Interventions:

TAKE ACTION

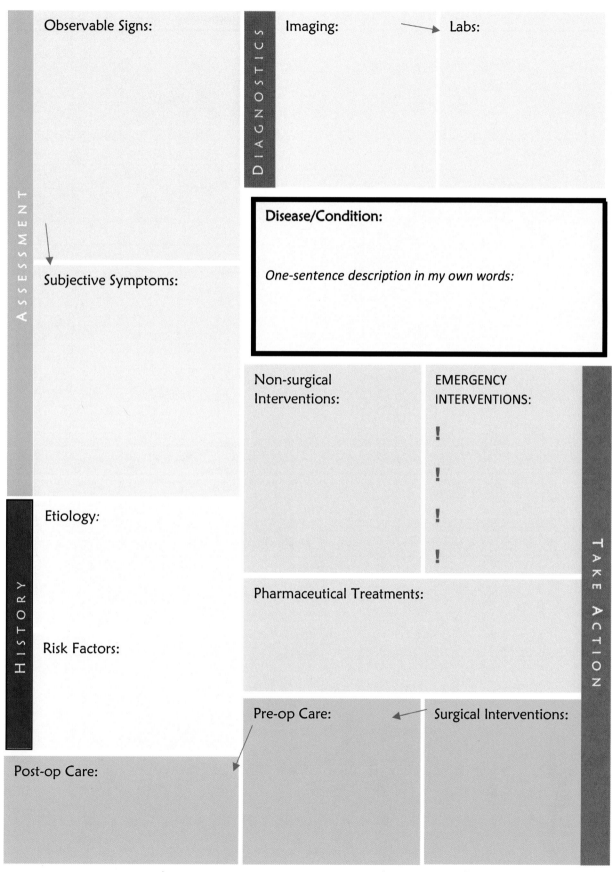

ASSESSMENT

Observable Signs:

Subjective Symptoms:

HISTORY

Etiology:

Risk Factors:

Post-op Care:

DIAGNOSTICS

Imaging:

Labs:

Disease/Condition:

One-sentence description in my own words:

Non-surgical Interventions:

EMERGENCY INTERVENTIONS:

!

!

!

!

Pharmaceutical Treatments:

Pre-op Care:

Surgical Interventions:

TAKE ACTION

Date:

Class:

This content will appear on Exam #:

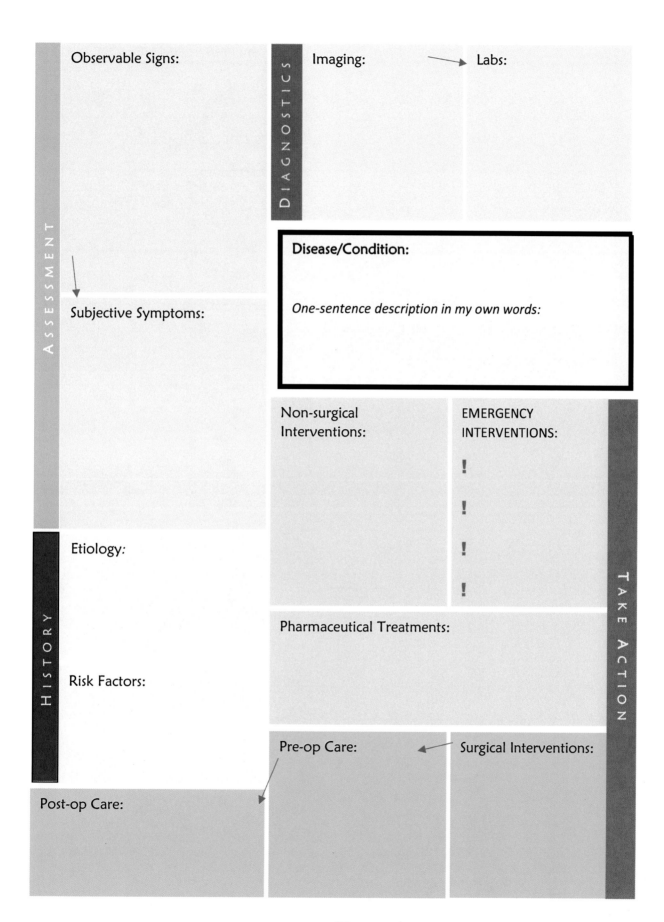

Observable Signs:

Imaging:

Labs:

ASSESSMENT

Subjective Symptoms:

Disease/Condition:

One-sentence description in my own words:

Non-surgical Interventions:

EMERGENCY INTERVENTIONS:

!

!

!

!

Etiology:

HISTORY

Pharmaceutical Treatments:

TAKE ACTION

Risk Factors:

Pre-op Care:

Surgical Interventions:

Post-op Care:

17

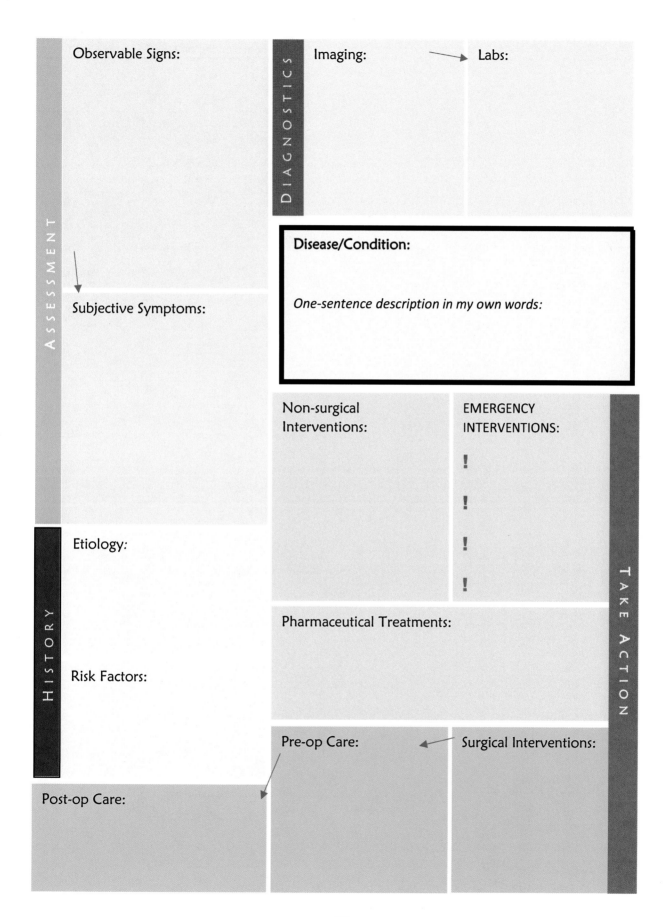

ASSESSMENT

Observable Signs:

Subjective Symptoms:

HISTORY

Etiology:

Risk Factors:

Post-op Care:

DIAGNOSTICS

Imaging:

Labs:

Disease/Condition:

One-sentence description in my own words:

Non-surgical
Interventions:

EMERGENCY
INTERVENTIONS:

!

!

!

!

Pharmaceutical Treatments:

Pre-op Care:

Surgical Interventions:

TAKE ACTION

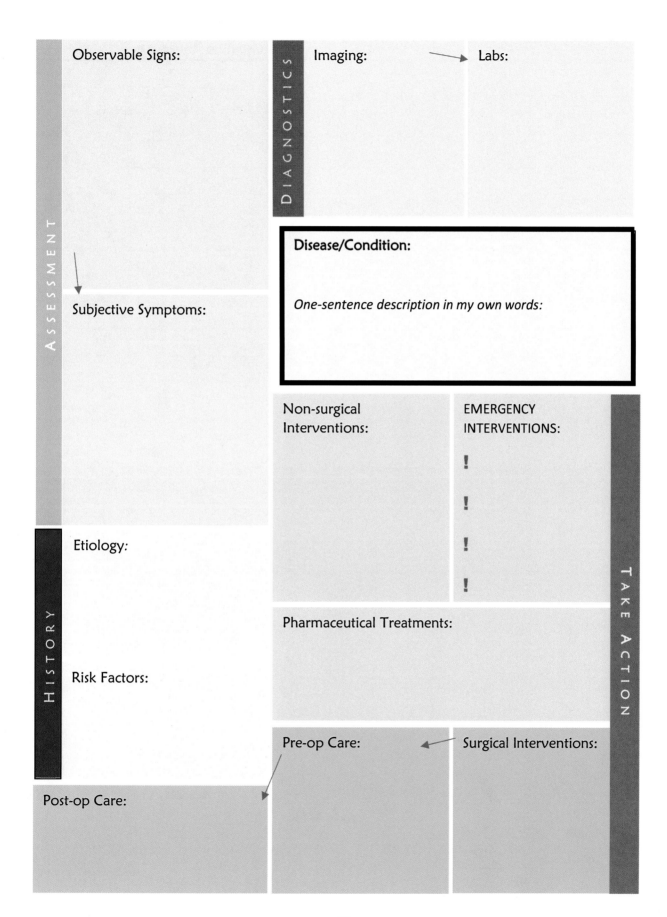

ASSESSMENT

Observable Signs:

Subjective Symptoms:

HISTORY

Etiology:

Risk Factors:

DIAGNOSTICS

Imaging:

Labs:

Disease/Condition:

One-sentence description in my own words:

TAKE ACTION

Non-surgical Interventions:

EMERGENCY INTERVENTIONS:

!

!

!

!

Pharmaceutical Treatments:

Pre-op Care:

Surgical Interventions:

Post-op Care:

Date: Class: This content will appear on Exam #:

22

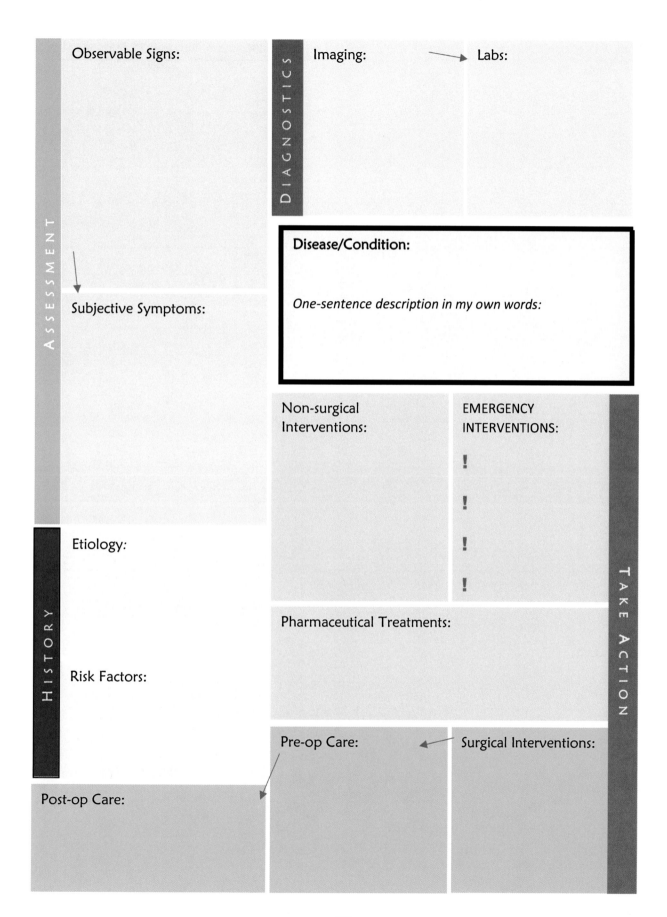

ASSESSMENT

Observable Signs:

Subjective Symptoms:

HISTORY

Etiology:

Risk Factors:

Post-op Care:

DIAGNOSTICS

Imaging:

Labs:

Disease/Condition:

One-sentence description in my own words:

Non-surgical Interventions:

EMERGENCY INTERVENTIONS:

!

!

!

!

Pharmaceutical Treatments:

Pre-op Care:

Surgical Interventions:

TAKE ACTION

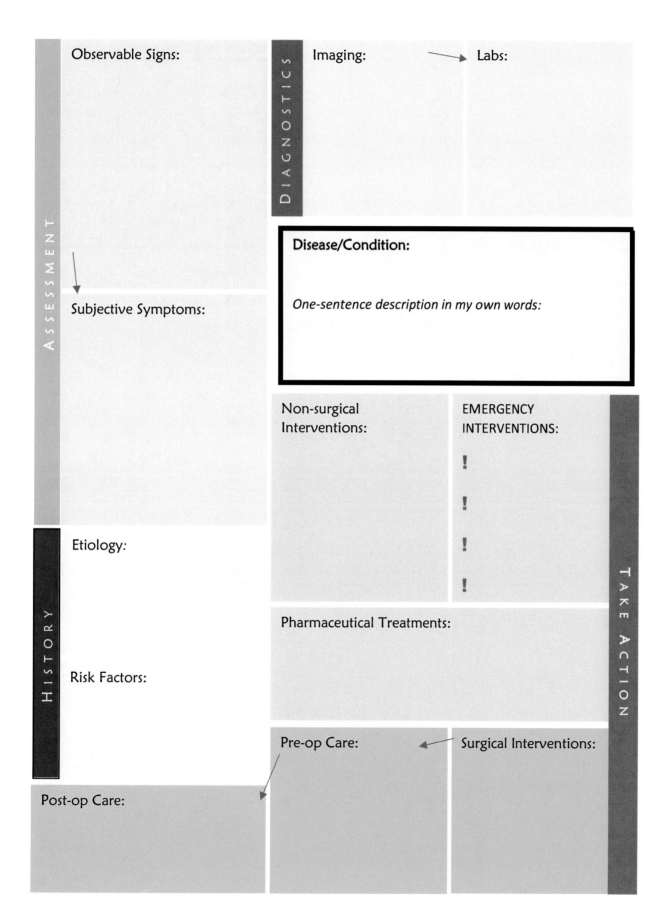

ASSESSMENT

Observable Signs:

Subjective Symptoms:

HISTORY

Etiology:

Risk Factors:

Post-op Care:

DIAGNOSTICS

Imaging:

Labs:

Disease/Condition:

One-sentence description in my own words:

Non-surgical Interventions:

EMERGENCY INTERVENTIONS:

!

!

!

!

Pharmaceutical Treatments:

Pre-op Care:

Surgical Interventions:

TAKE ACTION

Observable Signs:

DIAGNOSTICS

Imaging: Labs:

ASSESSMENT

Subjective Symptoms:

Disease/Condition:

One-sentence description in my own words:

Etiology:

Non-surgical
Interventions:

EMERGENCY
INTERVENTIONS:

!

!

!

!

HISTORY

Pharmaceutical Treatments:

TAKE ACTION

Risk Factors:

Pre-op Care: Surgical Interventions:

Post-op Care:

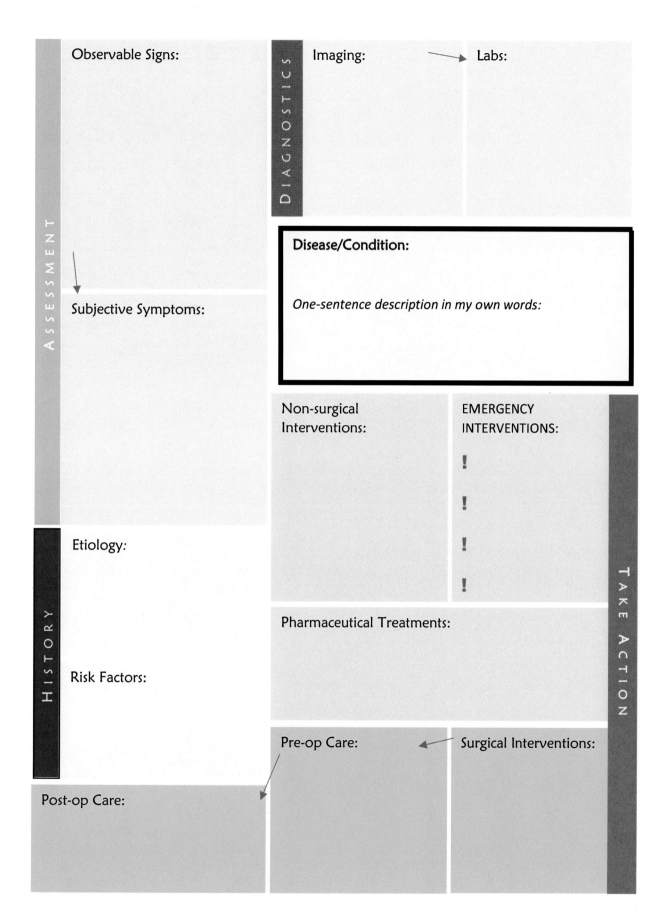

ASSESSMENT

Observable Signs:

Subjective Symptoms:

HISTORY

Etiology:

Risk Factors:

Post-op Care:

DIAGNOSTICS

Imaging:

Labs:

Disease/Condition:

One-sentence description in my own words:

Non-surgical Interventions:

EMERGENCY INTERVENTIONS:

!

!

!

!

Pharmaceutical Treatments:

Pre-op Care:

Surgical Interventions:

TAKE ACTION

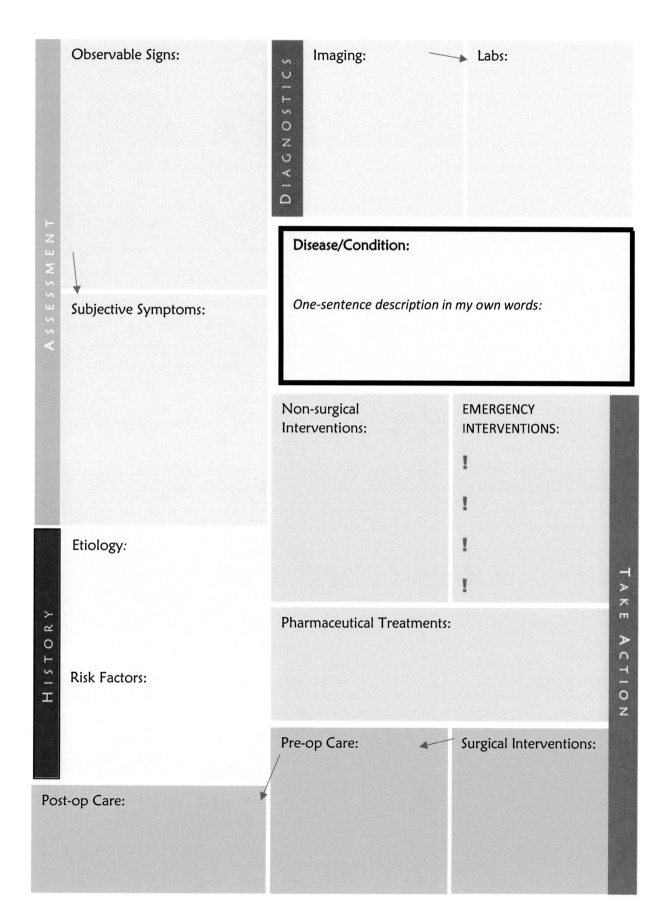

ASSESSMENT

Observable Signs:

Subjective Symptoms:

HISTORY

Etiology:

Risk Factors:

Post-op Care:

DIAGNOSTICS

Imaging:

Labs:

Disease/Condition:

One-sentence description in my own words:

Non-surgical Interventions:

EMERGENCY INTERVENTIONS:

!

!

!

!

Pharmaceutical Treatments:

Pre-op Care:

Surgical Interventions:

TAKE ACTION

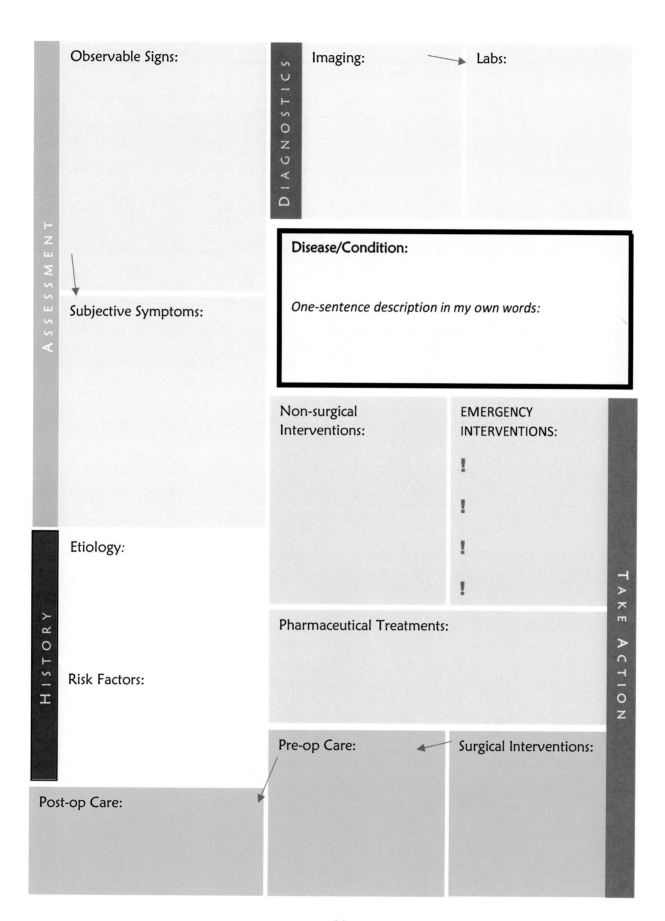

ASSESSMENT

Observable Signs:

Subjective Symptoms:

HISTORY

Etiology:

Risk Factors:

Post-op Care:

DIAGNOSTICS

Imaging:

Labs:

Disease/Condition:

One-sentence description in my own words:

Non-surgical Interventions:

EMERGENCY INTERVENTIONS:

!

!

!

!

Pharmaceutical Treatments:

Pre-op Care:

Surgical Interventions:

TAKE ACTION

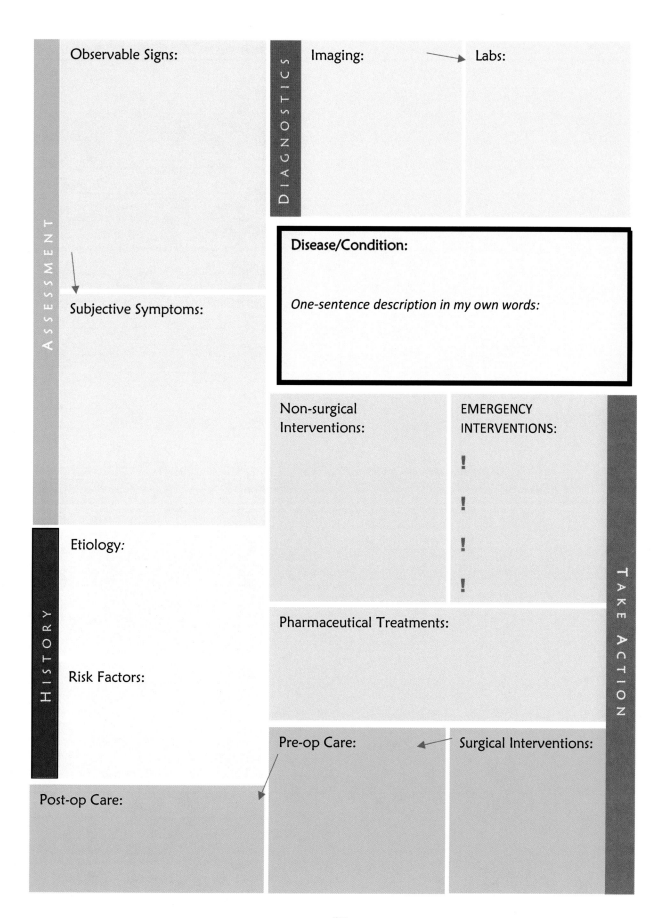

ASSESSMENT

Observable Signs:

Subjective Symptoms:

HISTORY

Etiology:

Risk Factors:

DIAGNOSTICS

Imaging:

Labs:

Disease/Condition:

One-sentence description in my own words:

Non-surgical Interventions:

EMERGENCY INTERVENTIONS:

!

!

!

!

Pharmaceutical Treatments:

Pre-op Care:

Surgical Interventions:

Post-op Care:

TAKE ACTION

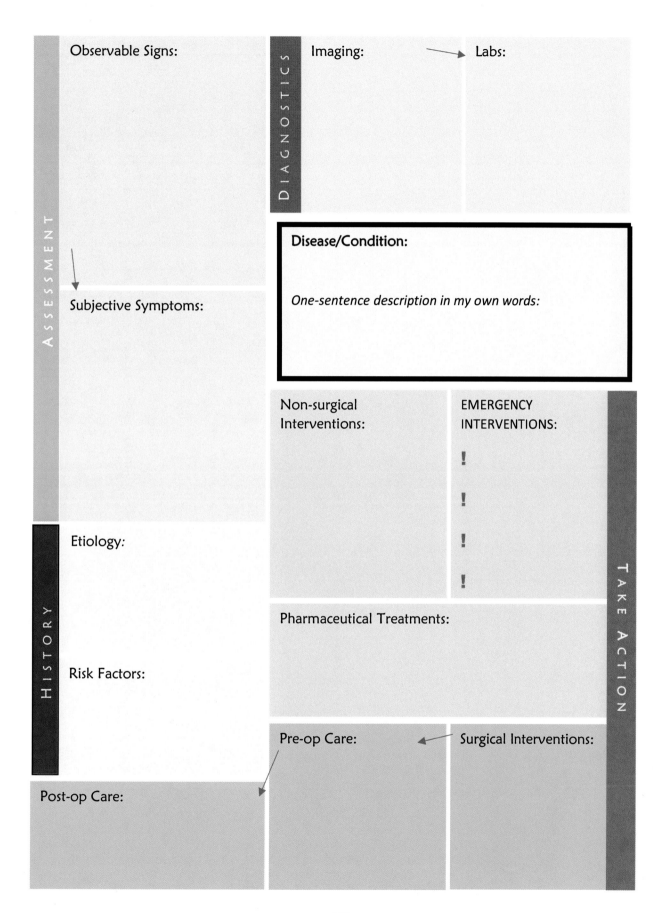

Observable Signs:

Imaging: → **Labs:**

DIAGNOSTICS

ASSESSMENT

Subjective Symptoms:

Disease/Condition:

One-sentence description in my own words:

Non-surgical Interventions:

EMERGENCY INTERVENTIONS:

!

!

!

!

Etiology:

HISTORY

Pharmaceutical Treatments:

TAKE ACTION

Risk Factors:

Pre-op Care: ← **Surgical Interventions:**

Post-op Care:

Date: Class: This content will appear on Exam #:

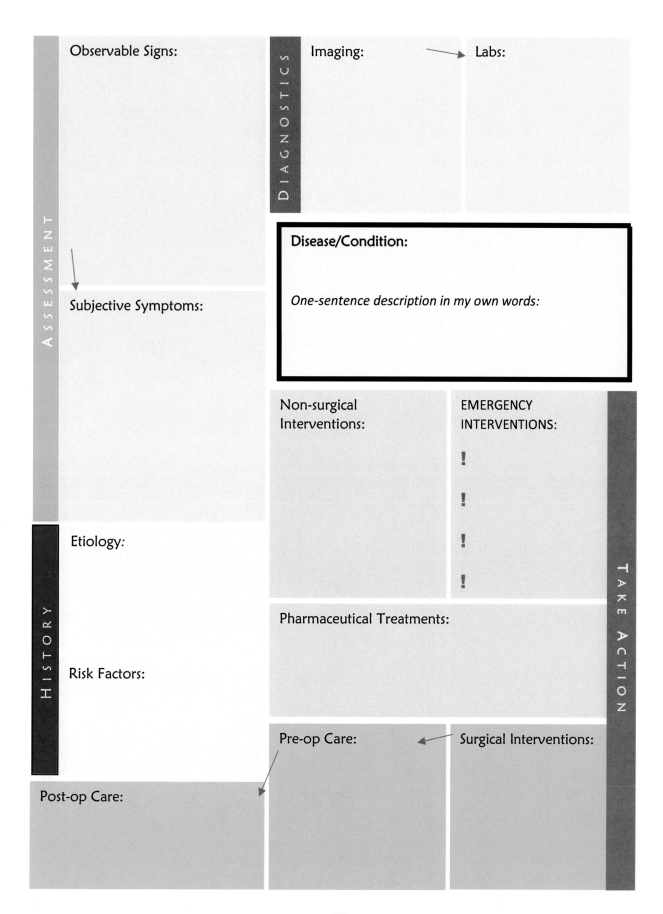

Observable Signs:

DIAGNOSTICS

Imaging:

Labs:

ASSESSMENT

Subjective Symptoms:

Disease/Condition:

One-sentence description in my own words:

Non-surgical
Interventions:

EMERGENCY
INTERVENTIONS:

!

!

!

!

HISTORY

Etiology:

Risk Factors:

Pharmaceutical Treatments:

TAKE ACTION

Pre-op Care:

Surgical Interventions:

Post-op Care:

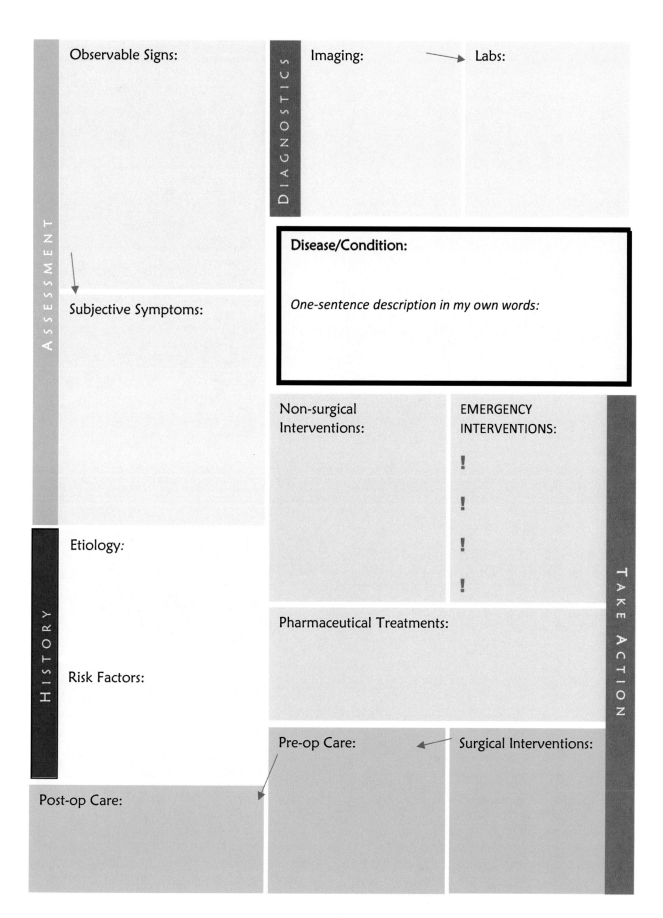

Observable Signs:

Imaging:

Labs:

DIAGNOSTICS

ASSESSMENT

Subjective Symptoms:

Disease/Condition:

One-sentence description in my own words:

Non-surgical
Interventions:

EMERGENCY
INTERVENTIONS:

!

!

!

!

Etiology:

HISTORY

Pharmaceutical Treatments:

TAKE ACTION

Risk Factors:

Pre-op Care:

Surgical Interventions:

Post-op Care:

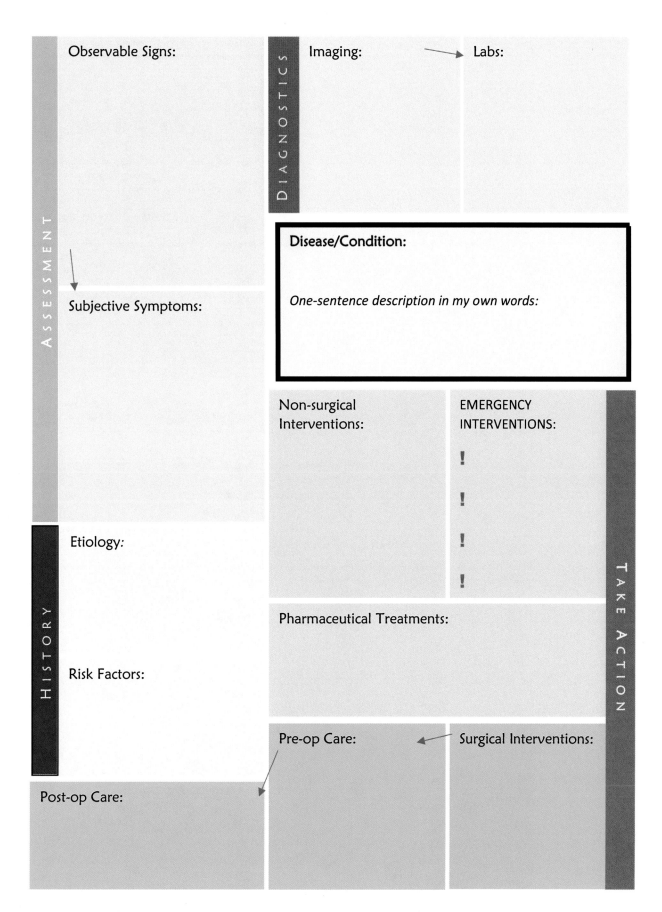

Observable Signs:

ASSESSMENT

Subjective Symptoms:

HISTORY

Etiology:

Risk Factors:

Post-op Care:

DIAGNOSTICS

Imaging:

Labs:

Disease/Condition:

One-sentence description in my own words:

Non-surgical Interventions:

EMERGENCY INTERVENTIONS:

!

!

!

!

Pharmaceutical Treatments:

Pre-op Care:

Surgical Interventions:

TAKE ACTION

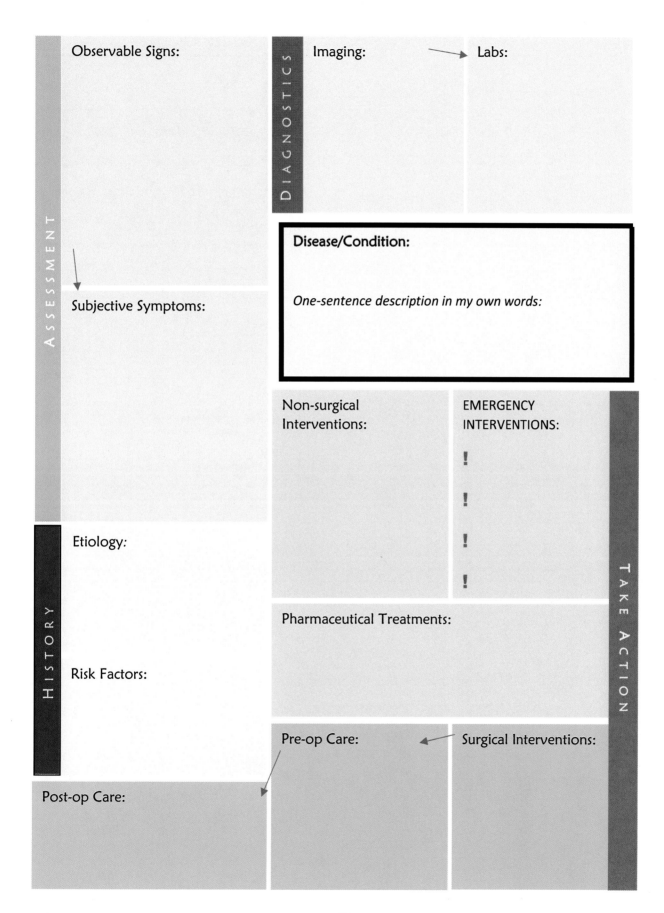

Observable Signs:

Imaging:

Labs:

DIAGNOSTICS

ASSESSMENT

Subjective Symptoms:

Disease/Condition:

One-sentence description in my own words:

Etiology:

Non-surgical Interventions:

EMERGENCY INTERVENTIONS:

!

!

!

!

HISTORY

TAKE ACTION

Pharmaceutical Treatments:

Risk Factors:

Pre-op Care:

Surgical Interventions:

Post-op Care:

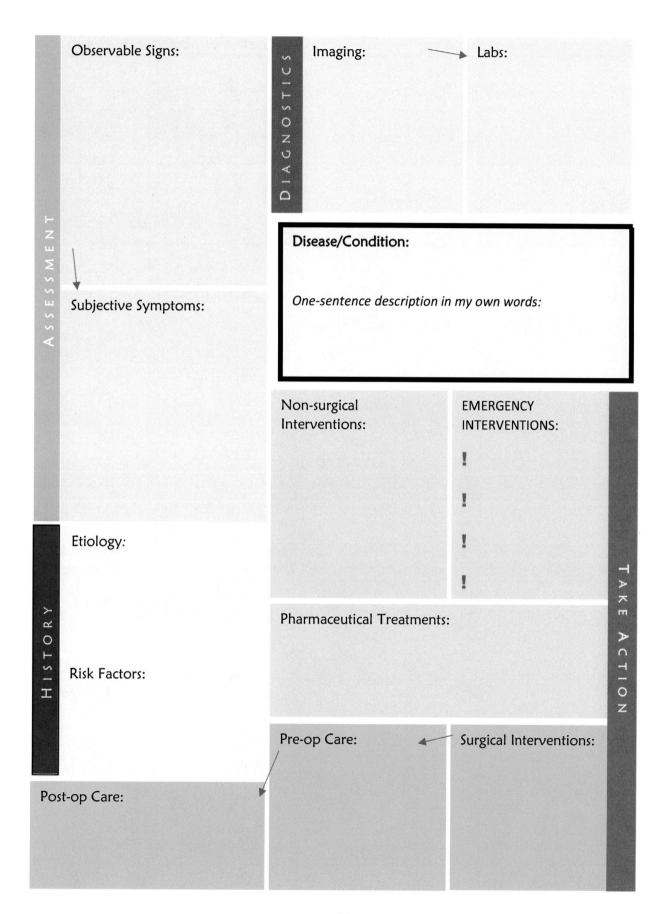

ASSESSMENT

Observable Signs:

Subjective Symptoms:

HISTORY

Etiology:

Risk Factors:

Post-op Care:

DIAGNOSTICS

Imaging:

Labs:

Disease/Condition:

One-sentence description in my own words:

Non-surgical Interventions:

EMERGENCY INTERVENTIONS:

!

!

!

!

Pharmaceutical Treatments:

Pre-op Care:

Surgical Interventions:

TAKE ACTION

47

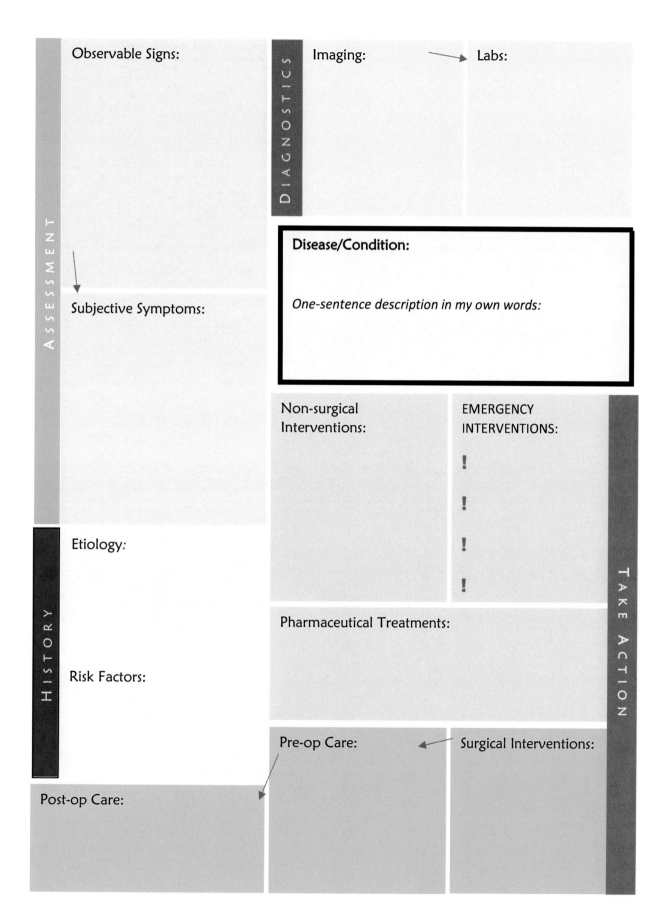

ASSESSMENT

Observable Signs:

Subjective Symptoms:

HISTORY

Etiology:

Risk Factors:

Post-op Care:

DIAGNOSTICS

Imaging:

Labs:

Disease/Condition:

One-sentence description in my own words:

Non-surgical Interventions:

EMERGENCY INTERVENTIONS:

!

!

!

!

Pharmaceutical Treatments:

Pre-op Care:

Surgical Interventions:

TAKE ACTION

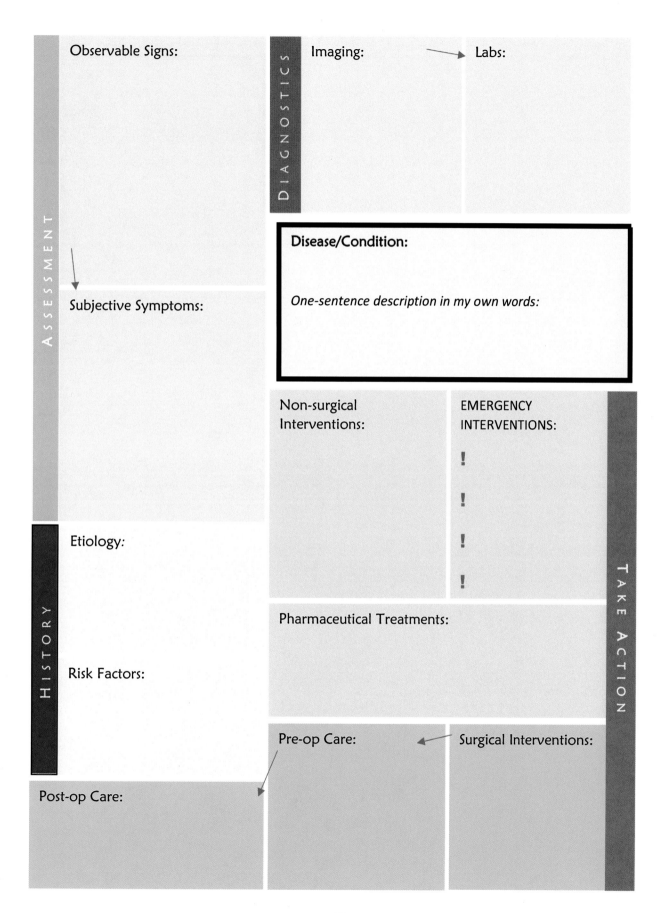

ASSESSMENT

Observable Signs:

Subjective Symptoms:

HISTORY

Etiology:

Risk Factors:

Post-op Care:

DIAGNOSTICS

Imaging:

Labs:

Disease/Condition:

One-sentence description in my own words:

Non-surgical Interventions:

EMERGENCY INTERVENTIONS:

!

!

!

!

Pharmaceutical Treatments:

Pre-op Care:

Surgical Interventions:

TAKE ACTION

Date: Class: This content will appear on Exam #:

Observable Signs:

DIAGNOSTICS

Imaging: Labs:

ASSESSMENT

Subjective Symptoms:

Disease/Condition:

One-sentence description in my own words:

Non-surgical
Interventions:

EMERGENCY
INTERVENTIONS:

!

!

!

!

HISTORY

Etiology:

Pharmaceutical Treatments:

Risk Factors:

TAKE ACTION

Pre-op Care: Surgical Interventions:

Post-op Care:

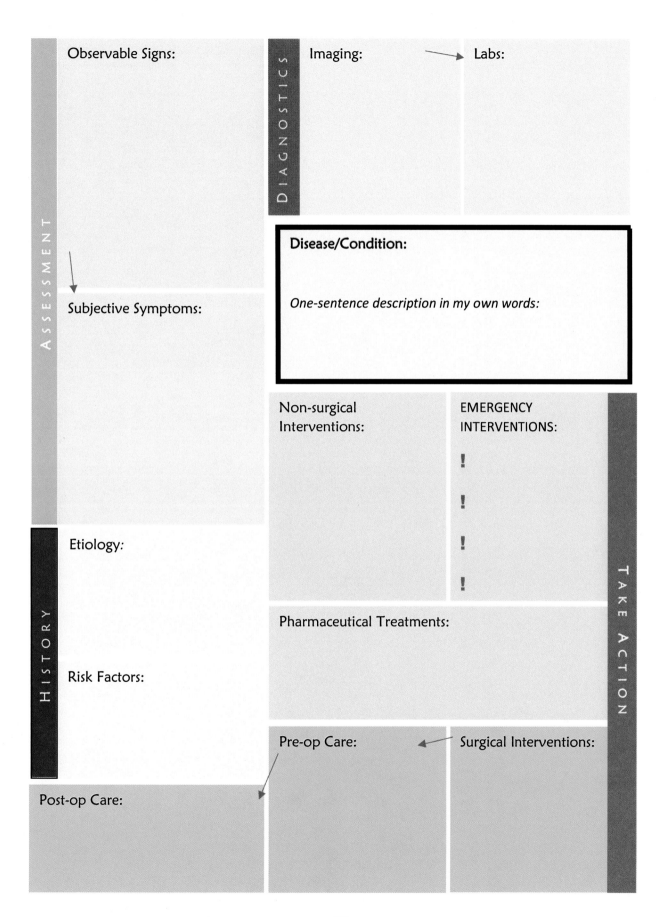

ASSESSMENT

Observable Signs:

Subjective Symptoms:

HISTORY

Etiology:

Risk Factors:

Post-op Care:

DIAGNOSTICS

Imaging:

Labs:

Disease/Condition:

One-sentence description in my own words:

Non-surgical Interventions:

EMERGENCY INTERVENTIONS:

!

!

!

!

Pharmaceutical Treatments:

Pre-op Care:

Surgical Interventions:

TAKE ACTION

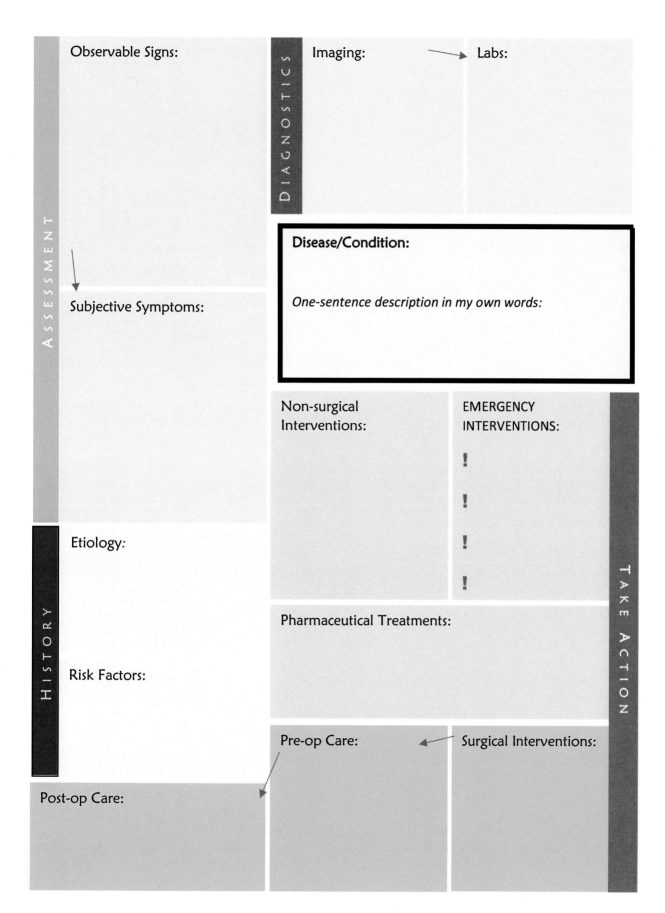

Observable Signs:

Imaging:

Labs:

ASSESSMENT

Subjective Symptoms:

Disease/Condition:

One-sentence description in my own words:

Non-surgical Interventions:

EMERGENCY INTERVENTIONS:

!

!

!

!

TAKE ACTION

Etiology:

HISTORY

Risk Factors:

Pharmaceutical Treatments:

Pre-op Care:

Surgical Interventions:

Post-op Care:

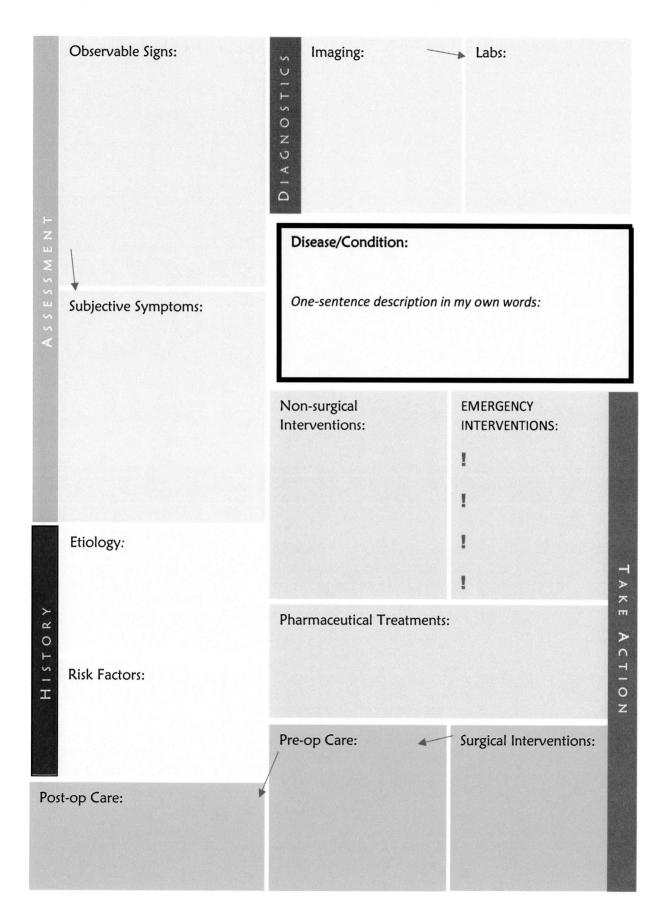

ASSESSMENT

Observable Signs:

Subjective Symptoms:

HISTORY

Etiology:

Risk Factors:

Post-op Care:

DIAGNOSTICS

Imaging:

Labs:

Disease/Condition:

One-sentence description in my own words:

Non-surgical Interventions:

EMERGENCY INTERVENTIONS:

!

!

!

!

Pharmaceutical Treatments:

Pre-op Care:

Surgical Interventions:

TAKE ACTION

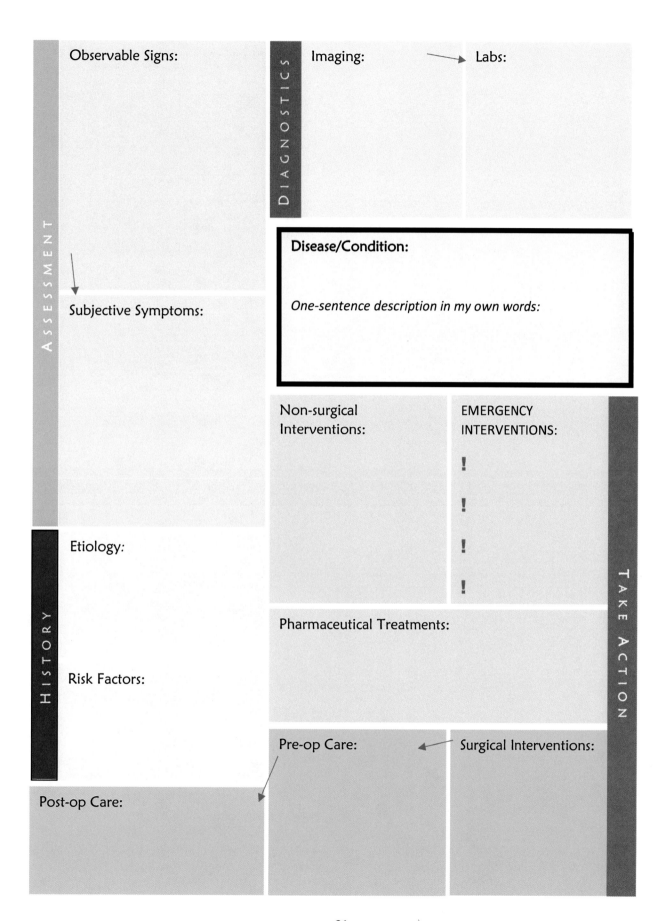

Observable Signs:

DIAGNOSTICS

Imaging:

Labs:

ASSESSMENT

Subjective Symptoms:

Disease/Condition:

One-sentence description in my own words:

Non-surgical
Interventions:

EMERGENCY
INTERVENTIONS:

!

!

!

!

HISTORY

Etiology:

Risk Factors:

Pharmaceutical Treatments:

TAKE ACTION

Pre-op Care:

Surgical Interventions:

Post-op Care:

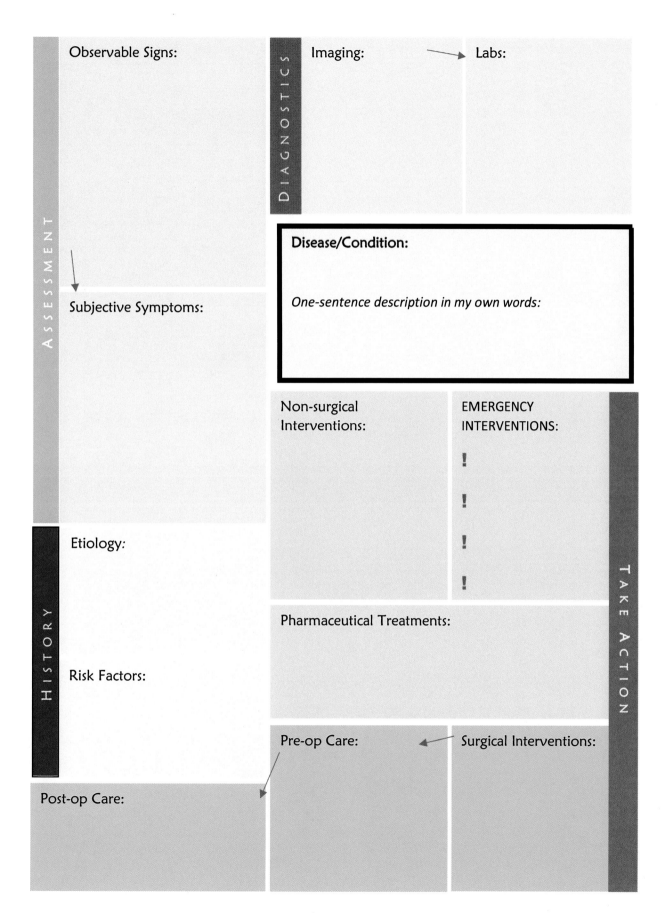

ASSESSMENT

Observable Signs:

Subjective Symptoms:

HISTORY

Etiology:

Risk Factors:

Post-op Care:

DIAGNOSTICS

Imaging:

Labs:

Disease/Condition:

One-sentence description in my own words:

Non-surgical Interventions:

EMERGENCY INTERVENTIONS:

!

!

!

!

Pharmaceutical Treatments:

Pre-op Care:

Surgical Interventions:

TAKE ACTION

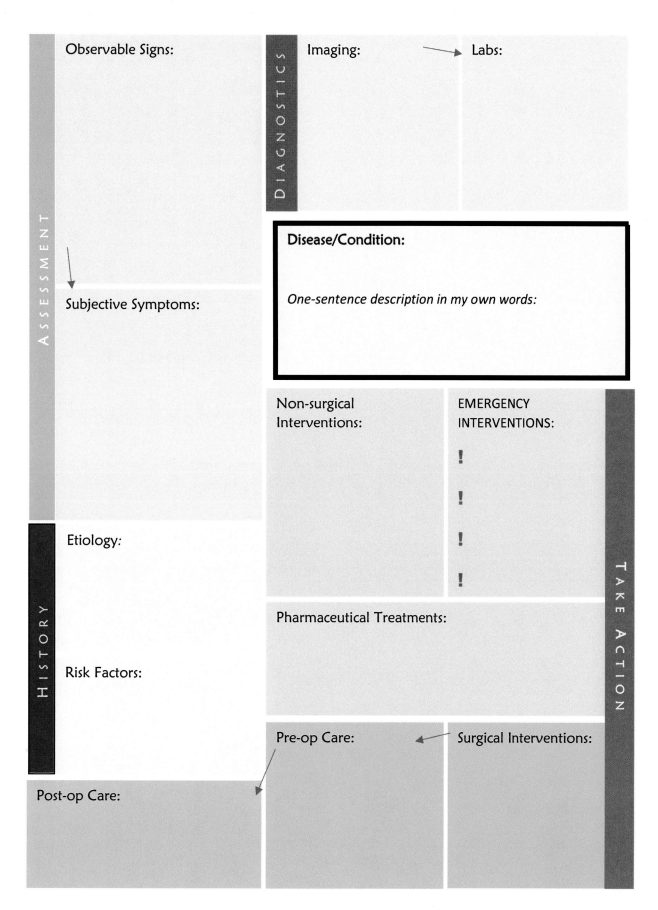

ASSESSMENT

Observable Signs:

Subjective Symptoms:

HISTORY

Etiology:

Risk Factors:

Post-op Care:

DIAGNOSTICS

Imaging:

Labs:

Disease/Condition:

One-sentence description in my own words:

Non-surgical
Interventions:

EMERGENCY
INTERVENTIONS:

!

!

!

!

Pharmaceutical Treatments:

Pre-op Care:

Surgical Interventions:

TAKE ACTION

Date: Class: This content will appear on Exam #:

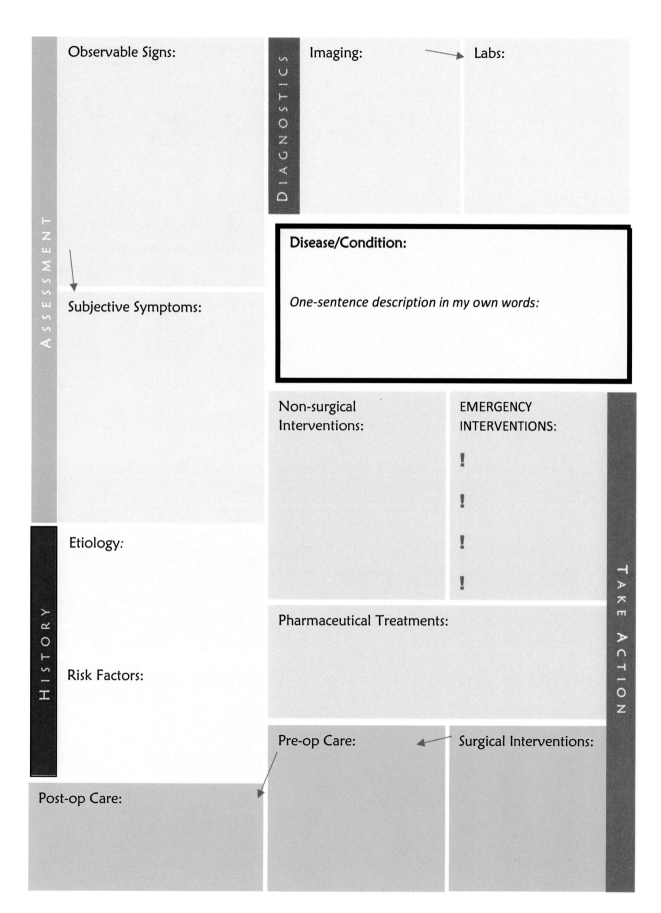

Observable Signs:

ASSESSMENT

DIAGNOSTICS

Imaging:

Labs:

Subjective Symptoms:

Disease/Condition:

One-sentence description in my own words:

Non-surgical
Interventions:

EMERGENCY
INTERVENTIONS:

!

!

!

!

HISTORY

Etiology:

Risk Factors:

Pharmaceutical Treatments:

TAKE ACTION

Pre-op Care:

Surgical Interventions:

Post-op Care:

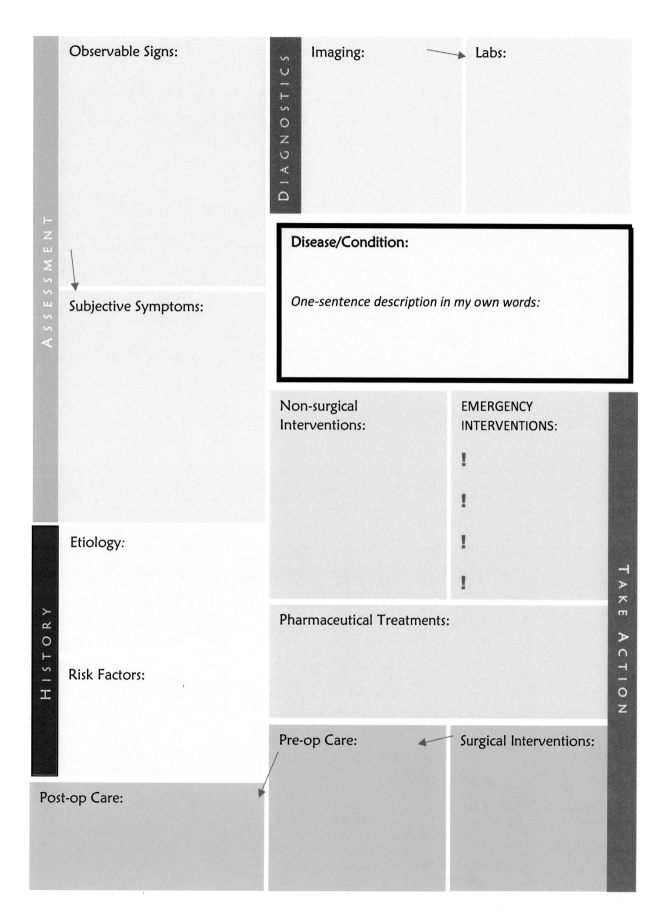

Observable Signs:

Imaging:

Labs:

DIAGNOSTICS

ASSESSMENT

Subjective Symptoms:

Disease/Condition:

One-sentence description in my own words:

Etiology:

Non-surgical Interventions:

EMERGENCY INTERVENTIONS:

!

!

!

!

Pharmaceutical Treatments:

HISTORY

Risk Factors:

TAKE ACTION

Pre-op Care:

Surgical Interventions:

Post-op Care:

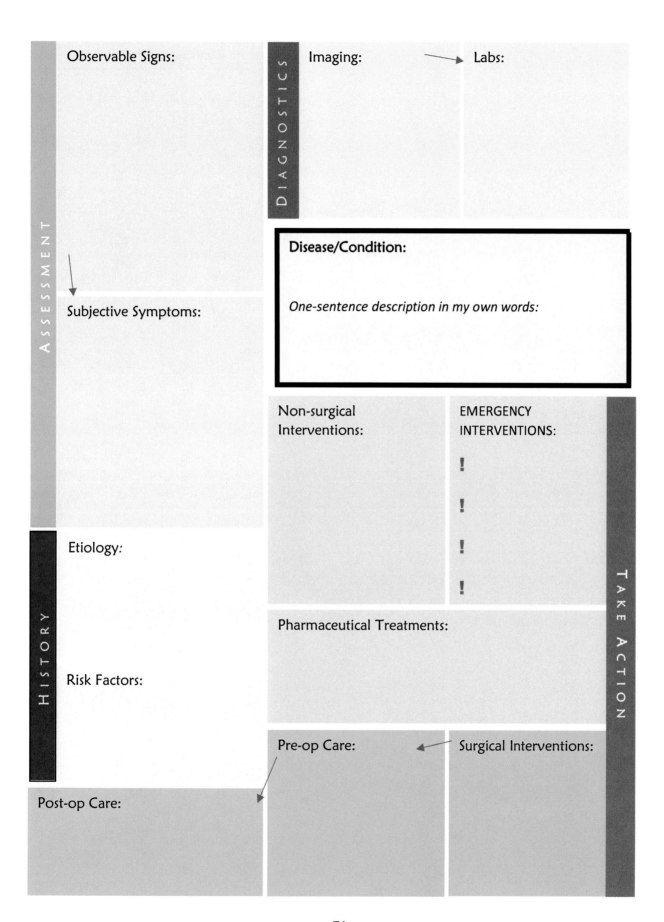

ASSESSMENT

Observable Signs:

DIAGNOSTICS

Imaging:

Labs:

Subjective Symptoms:

Disease/Condition:

One-sentence description in my own words:

HISTORY

Etiology:

Risk Factors:

Non-surgical
Interventions:

EMERGENCY
INTERVENTIONS:

!

!

!

!

Pharmaceutical Treatments:

TAKE ACTION

Pre-op Care:

Surgical Interventions:

Post-op Care:

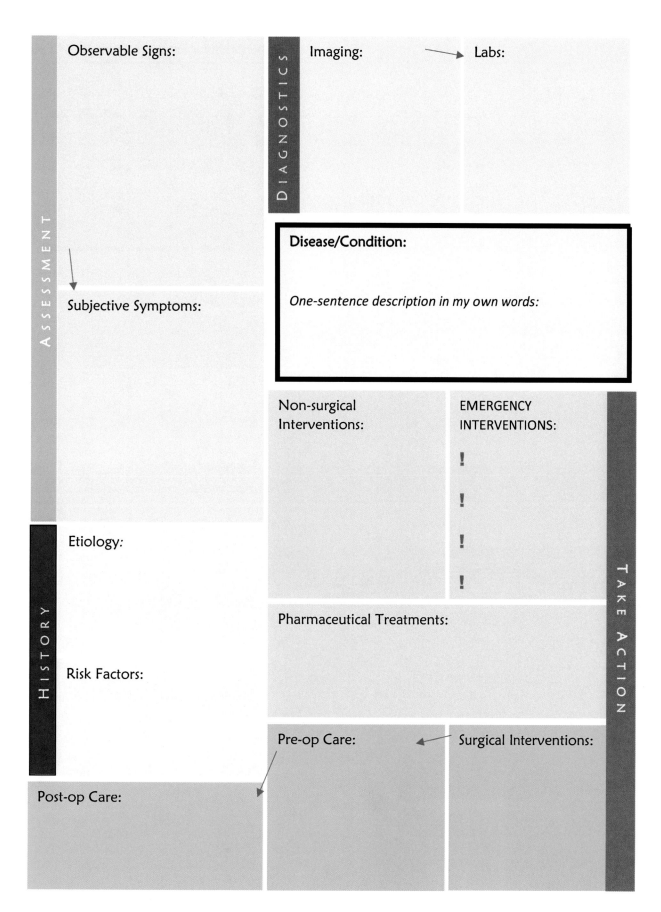

Observable Signs:

DIAGNOSTICS

Imaging:

Labs:

ASSESSMENT

Subjective Symptoms:

Disease/Condition:

One-sentence description in my own words:

Non-surgical Interventions:

EMERGENCY INTERVENTIONS:

!

!

!

!

TAKE ACTION

Etiology:

HISTORY

Pharmaceutical Treatments:

Risk Factors:

Pre-op Care:

Surgical Interventions:

Post-op Care:

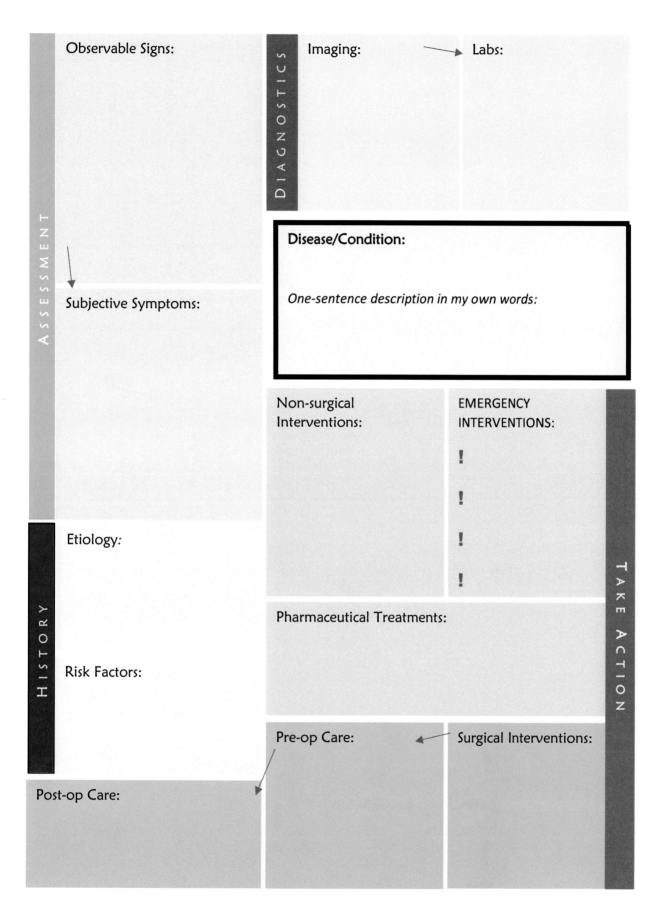

ASSESSMENT

Observable Signs:

Subjective Symptoms:

HISTORY

Etiology:

Risk Factors:

Post-op Care:

DIAGNOSTICS

Imaging:

Labs:

Disease/Condition:

One-sentence description in my own words:

Non-surgical Interventions:

EMERGENCY INTERVENTIONS:

!

!

!

!

Pharmaceutical Treatments:

Pre-op Care:

Surgical Interventions:

TAKE ACTION

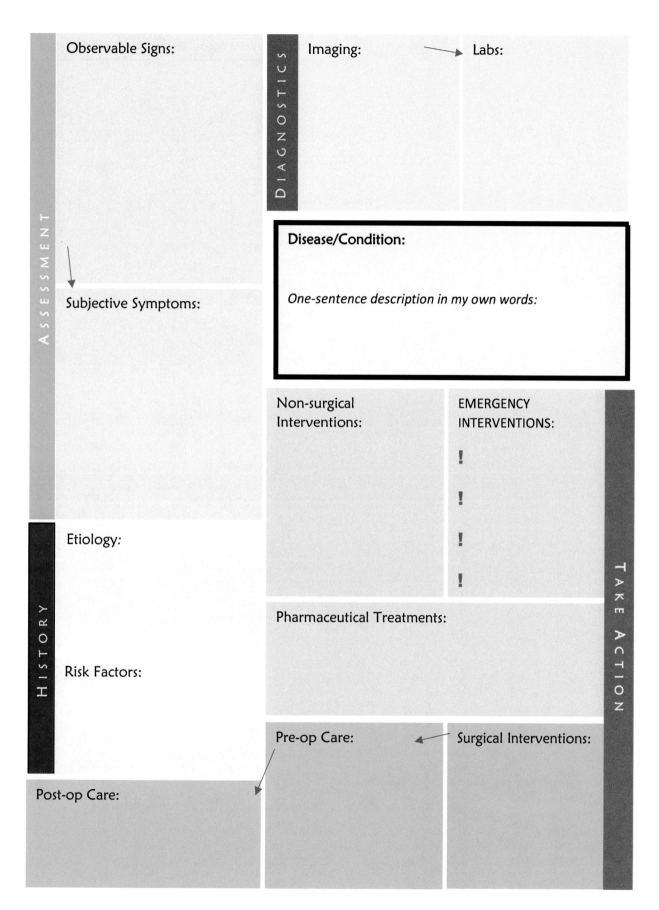

Observable Signs:

Imaging:

Labs:

Subjective Symptoms:

Disease/Condition:

One-sentence description in my own words:

Non-surgical Interventions:

EMERGENCY INTERVENTIONS:

!

!

!

!

Etiology:

Risk Factors:

Pharmaceutical Treatments:

Pre-op Care:

Surgical Interventions:

Post-op Care:

77

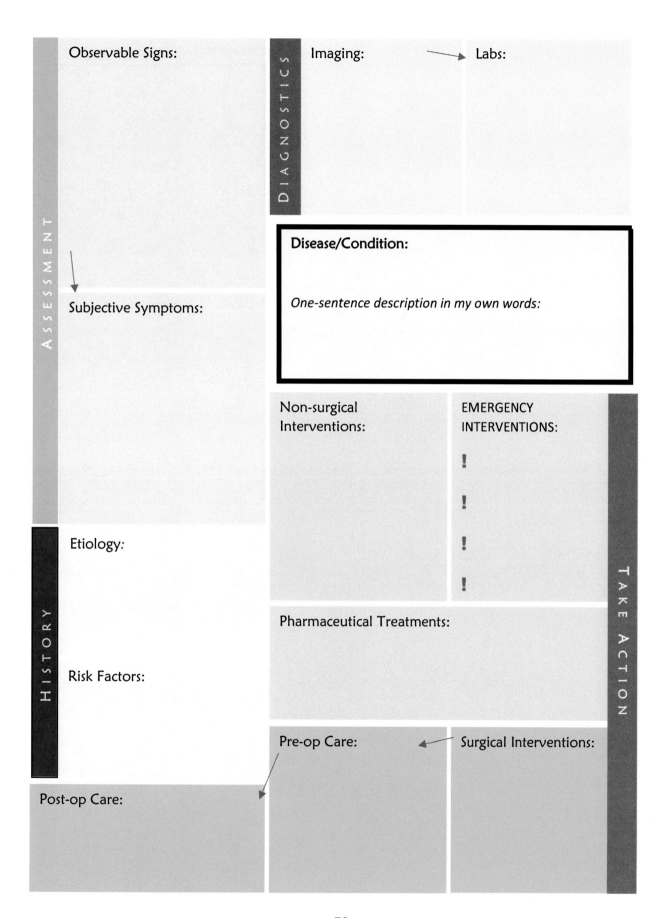

ASSESSMENT

Observable Signs:

Subjective Symptoms:

HISTORY

Etiology:

Risk Factors:

Post-op Care:

DIAGNOSTICS

Imaging:

Labs:

Disease/Condition:

One-sentence description in my own words:

Non-surgical
Interventions:

EMERGENCY
INTERVENTIONS:

!

!

!

!

Pharmaceutical Treatments:

Pre-op Care:

Surgical Interventions:

TAKE ACTION

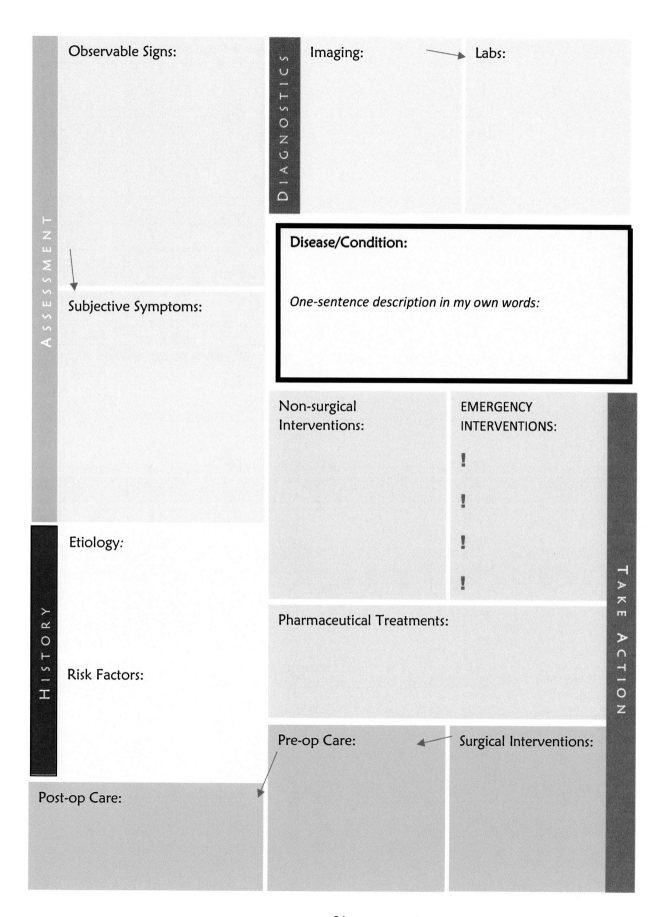

ASSESSMENT

Observable Signs:

Subjective Symptoms:

HISTORY

Etiology:

Risk Factors:

Post-op Care:

DIAGNOSTICS

Imaging:

Labs:

Disease/Condition:

One-sentence description in my own words:

Non-surgical Interventions:

EMERGENCY INTERVENTIONS:

!

!

!

!

Pharmaceutical Treatments:

Pre-op Care:

Surgical Interventions:

TAKE ACTION

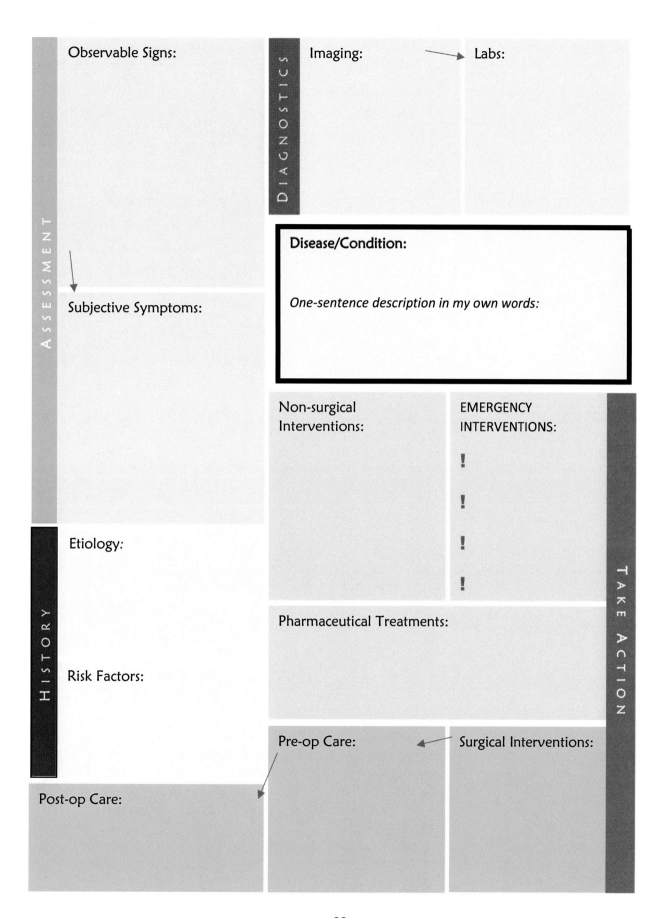

Observable Signs:

ASSESSMENT

Subjective Symptoms:

HISTORY

Etiology:

Risk Factors:

DIAGNOSTICS

Imaging:

Labs:

Disease/Condition:

One-sentence description in my own words:

Non-surgical
Interventions:

EMERGENCY
INTERVENTIONS:

!

!

!

!

Pharmaceutical Treatments:

TAKE ACTION

Pre-op Care:

Surgical Interventions:

Post-op Care:

Observable Signs:

Imaging:

Labs:

Subjective Symptoms:

Disease/Condition:

One-sentence description in my own words:

Etiology:

Non-surgical Interventions:

EMERGENCY INTERVENTIONS:

!

!

!

!

Pharmaceutical Treatments:

Risk Factors:

Pre-op Care:

Surgical Interventions:

Post-op Care:

Observable Signs:

Imaging:

Labs:

ASSESSMENT

Subjective Symptoms:

Disease/Condition:

One-sentence description in my own words:

Non-surgical
Interventions:

EMERGENCY
INTERVENTIONS:

!

!

!

!

Etiology:

TAKE ACTION

Pharmaceutical Treatments:

HISTORY

Risk Factors:

Pre-op Care:

Surgical Interventions:

Post-op Care:

Observable Signs:

DIAGNOSTICS

Imaging:

Labs:

ASSESSMENT

Subjective Symptoms:

Disease/Condition:

One-sentence description in my own words:

Non-surgical
Interventions:

EMERGENCY
INTERVENTIONS:

!

!

!

!

Etiology:

TAKE ACTION

Pharmaceutical Treatments:

HISTORY

Risk Factors:

Pre-op Care:

Surgical Interventions:

Post-op Care:

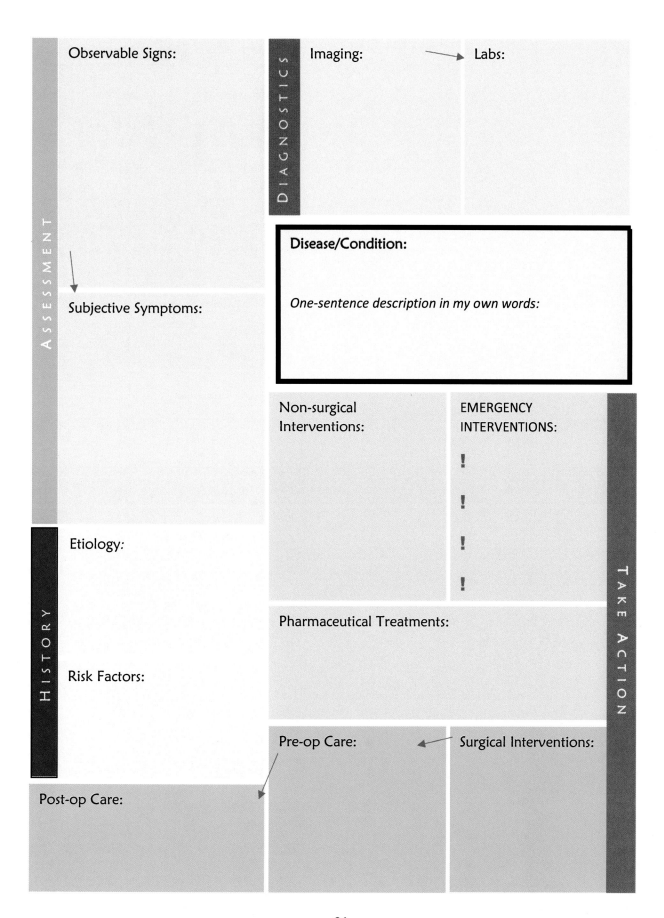

ASSESSMENT

Observable Signs:

Subjective Symptoms:

HISTORY

Etiology:

Risk Factors:

DIAGNOSTICS

Imaging:

Labs:

Disease/Condition:

One-sentence description in my own words:

Non-surgical Interventions:

EMERGENCY INTERVENTIONS:

!

!

!

!

Pharmaceutical Treatments:

Pre-op Care:

Surgical Interventions:

TAKE ACTION

Post-op Care:

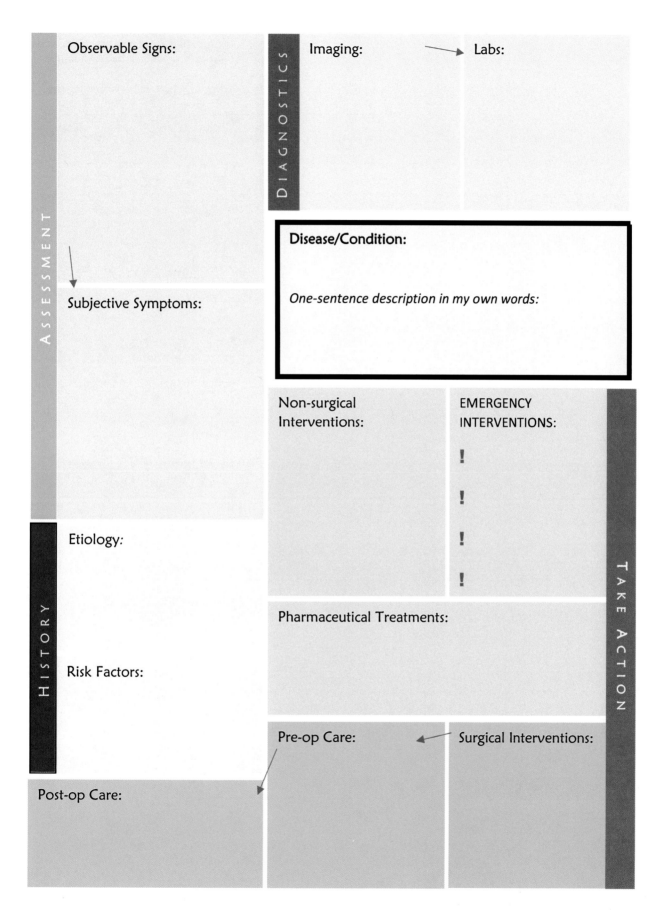

Observable Signs:

ASSESSMENT

Subjective Symptoms:

HISTORY

Etiology:

Risk Factors:

Post-op Care:

DIAGNOSTICS

Imaging:

Labs:

Disease/Condition:

One-sentence description in my own words:

Non-surgical Interventions:

EMERGENCY INTERVENTIONS:

!

!

!

!

Pharmaceutical Treatments:

Pre-op Care:

Surgical Interventions:

TAKE ACTION

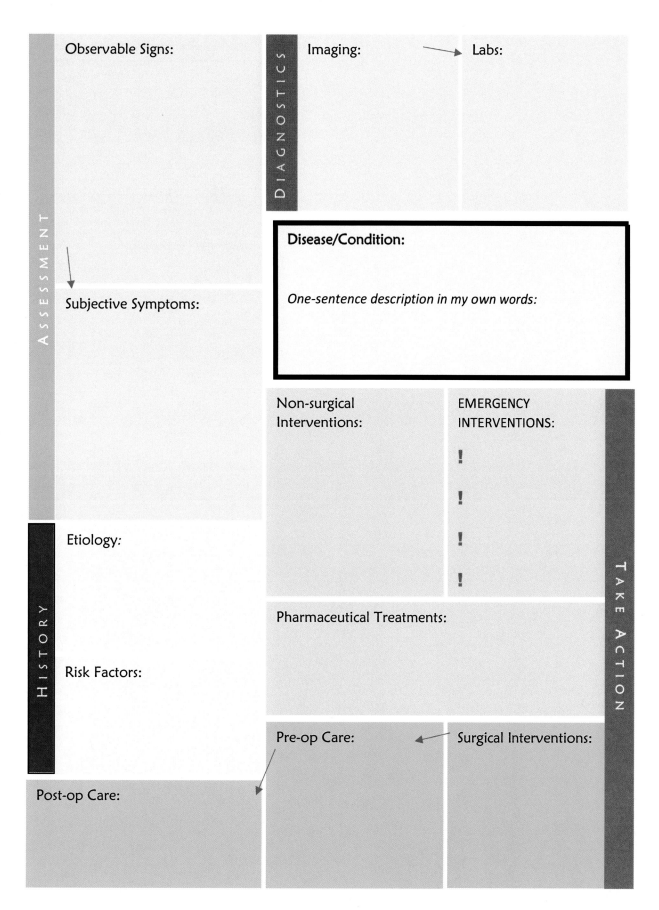

ASSESSMENT

Observable Signs:

Subjective Symptoms:

HISTORY

Etiology:

Risk Factors:

DIAGNOSTICS

Imaging:

Labs:

Disease/Condition:

One-sentence description in my own words:

Non-surgical Interventions:

EMERGENCY INTERVENTIONS:

!

!

!

!

Pharmaceutical Treatments:

Pre-op Care:

Surgical Interventions:

Post-op Care:

TAKE ACTION

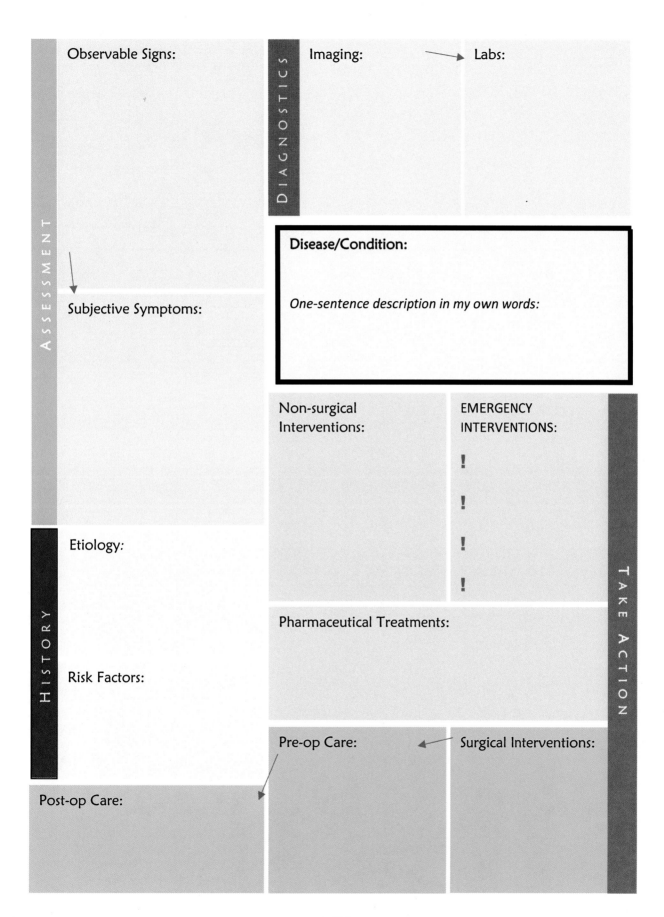

ASSESSMENT

Observable Signs:

Subjective Symptoms:

HISTORY

Etiology:

Risk Factors:

Post-op Care:

DIAGNOSTICS

Imaging:

Labs:

Disease/Condition:

One-sentence description in my own words:

Non-surgical
Interventions:

EMERGENCY
INTERVENTIONS:

!

!

!

!

Pharmaceutical Treatments:

Pre-op Care:

Surgical Interventions:

TAKE ACTION

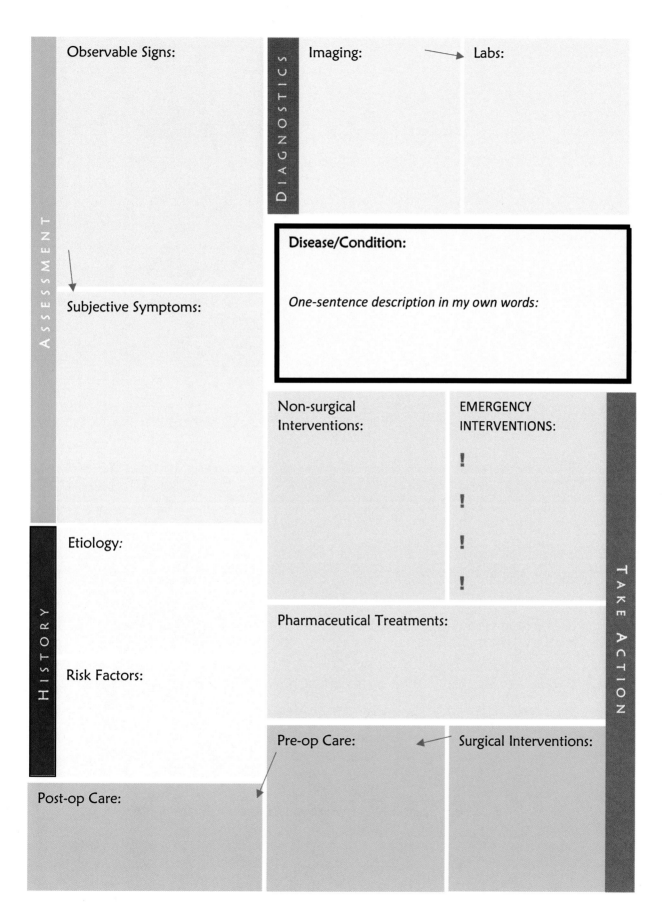

Observable Signs:

ASSESSMENT

DIAGNOSTICS

Imaging:

Labs:

Subjective Symptoms:

Disease/Condition:

One-sentence description in my own words:

HISTORY

Etiology:

Risk Factors:

Non-surgical
Interventions:

EMERGENCY
INTERVENTIONS:

!

!

!

!

TAKE ACTION

Pharmaceutical Treatments:

Pre-op Care:

Surgical Interventions:

Post-op Care:

Content I missed on unit exams that I need to review for the final:

Content I missed on unit exams that I need to review for the final:

Content I missed on unit exams that I need to review for the final:

Made in United States
Orlando, FL
25 May 2022

18191767R00058